Preg

Tariku E. Alemu

Pregnancy and Antenatal Care Service

Assessment of Late entry to antenatal care and its predictors among ANC attendees in Gambella Region, Ethiopia

LAP LAMBERT Academic Publishing

Imprint

Cover image: www.ingimage.com

Publisher:
LAP LAMBERT Academic Publishing
is a trademark of
International Book Market Service Ltd., member of OmniScriptum Publishing Group
17 Meldrum Street, Beau Bassin 71504, Mauritius

Printed at: see last page
ISBN: 978-613-9-96699-8

Acknowledgements

I wish to give glory and praise to the Almighty who gave me a good health, strength, courage and commitment to complete this thesis.

Many thanks for Addis Ababa University, School of public health for the financial assistance, without which the completion of the thesis would have been impossible.

I am also grateful to the following persons:

Professor Misganaw Fantahun, my advisor and promoter, for his unwavering support, encouragement and his preparedness to guide and share his knowledge and expertise with me.

The participants, for providing the required information for the study, data collectors and supervisors for their cooperation during period of data collection

My thanks also goes to Gambella Regional health bureau, Gambella hospital, Pugnudo health center, Abobo health center, and Metti health center for allowing me to conduct the study in the health facilities.

My heartfelt gratitude go to my father, mother, brothers, and sisters for their moral and material supports and engagements, without whom it would have been difficult to complete my study and thesis work.

Tables of contents

Page

Lists of tables and figures page

Lists of abbreviations

AAU	Addis Ababa University
ANC	Antenatal care
AOR	Adjusted Odds Ratio
CI	Confidence Interval
CSA	Central Statistical Authority
COR	Crude Odds Ratio
EDHS	Ethiopian Demographic and Health Survey
FGD	Focus Group Discussion
FMoH	Federal Ministry of Health
FoM	Faculty of Medicine
H/C	Health Center
IRB	Institutional Review Board
MCH	Maternal and Child Health
OR	Odds Ratio
RHB	Regional health Bureau
SPH	School of Public Health
SPSS	Statistical Package for Social Sciences
WHO	World Health Organization

Abstract

Background: *Antenatal care is more beneficial in preventing adverse pregnancy outcomes when it is sought early in the pregnancy and continued through to delivery. Despite the widespread availability of free antenatal care services, most women in our country attend their first antenatal clinic late in pregnancy and fail to return for follow up care, which potentially leads to perinatal and maternal complications.*

Objective: *The objective of the study is to assess late antenatal care booking and its predictors among pregnant women attending antenatal care in selected public health institution in Gambella Region, South West of Ethiopia.*

Methods: *Facility based crossectional study was conducted from March 15 to April 30, 2010 on selected samples 302 pregnant women attending antenatal care. Data were, collected through pretested structured questionnaire, entered in to Epi-info version 3.4 and then exported to SPSS-15 windows statistical packages for analysis. Bivariate and multivariate logistic regression was employed in order to infer associations and predictions.*

Result: *Forty eight percent of women commenced ANC after 16 weeks of gestation. The mean gestational age at booking was 4.6±1.4 months. When the effects of other independent variables on gestational age at booking were controlled, the following characteristics were found to be predictive of failure to initiate antenatal care by 16 weeks of gestation ($P<0.05$): unplanned pregnancy [AOR=2.85,95%CI (1.274,6.355)], past booking experience of antenatal care after 16weeks of gestation[AOR=5.85,95%CI(2.665,12.83)], reason for booking was thought the time was appropriate[AOR=2.15,95%CI(1.052,4.38)].*

Conclusion: *A significant proportion of mothers commenced antenatal care after 16 weeks of gestation in their pregnancies. It is concluded that unplanned pregnancy and the above two factors were a predictive of late entry to antenatal care in Gambella. These findings indicate that the importance of early antenatal booking is yet to be promoted.*

1. Introduction

The purpose of ANC is to improve pregnancy outcome for both the mother and fetus. To achieve this objective, the service is organized into a booking (first visit) and a follow up clinic. The aims and objectives of the first visits are primarily to establish a rapport with the client and collect information to evaluate the state of health of the mother, and her preparedness for motherhood and chart the likely course of the pregnancy. Early entry to antenatal care (ANC) is important for early detection and treatment of adverse pregnancy related outcomes(1, 2). A key objective of maternal health care programmes has been to ensure that women present for antenatal care early in pregnancy in order to allow enough time for essential diagnosis and treatment regimens such as treatment of STIs and management of anemia. The World Health Organization (WHO) recommends that pregnant women in developing countries should seek ANC within the first 4 months of pregnancy (1). In Ethiopia, according to EDHS 2005, only 6 percent of women make their first ANC visit before the fourth month of pregnancy (3).

1.1 Statement of the problem

Despite the facts that antenatal care is provided free of payment and physically accessible to most of pregnant women, majority of them are booking late to utilize the service.

This situation contributes to an increase in pregnant women's chance of infant and maternal morbidity and mortality. From the point of view of prenatal screening and complication prevention components of antenatal care, those pregnant women who booked after the recommended period of booking time are not benefiting from early pregnancy screening and counseling.

There is a general lack of both quantitative and qualitative research which addresses the phenomenon of late antenatal attendance or non-attendance. In addition to this, there is little knowledge on factors related to late entry to antenatal care and its predictors in Ethiopia in general and in Gambella region in particular.

It is against this background that the study was undertaken to examine late entry to prenatal care and its predictors among pregnant women in Gambella Region, South west of Ethiopia.

1.2 The significance of the study

Effective utilization of antenatal care service, through early booking for antenatal care, receiving health promotion information and health care, is crucial in enhancing maternal and fetal health during pregnancy and reducing maternal mortality and morbidity.

The identified predicting factors for late entry to antenatal care in the study area are envisaged to assist in:

1. Promoting quality antenatal care through evidence based practices
2. Enhance effective utilization of antenatal care by pregnant mothers in the region.
3. Bridging the information gap, and subsequently increase the number of early initiators of antenatal care in the region.
4. Planning and implementing antenatal care service utilization in the region.

2. Literature Review

Joint report from WHO and UNICEF on ANC in developing countries, pointed out that pregnant women in Sub-Saharan Africa who have started the first ANC within three months of pregnancy [during first trimester] are only about 20% which is least compared to other developing countries (1). Community based study done in Addis Ababa, reported that the proportion of women started their ANC checkup during the first trimester were only 26% (4).

According to Andersen health care seeking behavior model, health seeking behaviour is the result of interaction between characteristics of individuals, population and the surrounding environment. The model consists of several main components: predisposing characteristics (e.g. age, race), enabling resources (e.g. health insurance), needs (e.g. being sick or having further complications), personal health care behavior (e.g. exercise), outcomes (e.g. satisfaction with the health services) and environment (e.g. health care policies). The model has been widely used in studying factors related to utilization of different health care services (5).

Studies done on late antenatal care booking are limited. However, few studies available from different area reported the factors contributing for delayed initiation of antenatal care deferentially.

2.1 Predisposing factors

Maternal age

Younger and older women are different in their usage of maternal health services. Younger women tended to enter ANC later than older women. In a study conducted in Australia, 56% of women in their teens entered ANC late while only 36% of women in their 30's entered ANC late (6). Many studies reveal that teenagers are most likely to initiate late or no prenatal care (7-9).

Marital status

Married women are different in early initiation of prenatal care from that of unmarried once. In Finland, non attendance and under utilization of antenatal care were prevalent among unmarried women than married (8). In other studies it has been shown that married women were 40% more likely to receive antenatal care than unmarried women (10).

Maternal Education

Many studies indicated that maternal education is highly associated with early initiation of antenatal care (11, 12). In a study conducted in south west Nigerian pregnant women, those who had primary school education or none, 152(85.4%) were more likely to register late compared to those who had secondary school education and above, 215(79.3%), $p < 0.05$(9).

Occupation

Employed mothers had earlier booking and more visits than housewives (11, 13, 14). In other studies women with unemployed partners were, however, significantly more likely to book late for antenatal care than women with partners in employment(15).

Ethnicity and Religion

Compared with white women, black women were 1.7 times more likely to initiate prenatal care late or not at all when other study variables were controlled (7). A disturbing delay by all ethnic groups in the timing of their first antenatal visit was observed in Amsterdam. According to this finding all non-Dutch ethnic groups were significantly later in starting antenatal care during the whole duration of pregnancy compared with Dutch ethnicity (16).

A study on use of maternal health care service in Ethiopia showed that those women who followed Orthodox, Muslim and Protestant religions exhibited comparable and higher use of antenatal care (24.8- 28.3%), than those women who followed traditional beliefs (11.3%)(10).

2.2 Enabling factors

Place of residence

Being an urban or rural residence can significantly determine the use maternal health. Generally urban dwellers are more likely utilize ANC than the rural (1). In Ethiopia, finding form analysis of EDHS, 2005, identified that, place of residence was found one of the determinant factors for maternal health service utilization (3). In addition to this finding, a community based survey in southern Ethiopia, showed that there was a great difference in utilization of ANC service and timing of booking among urban and rural residents (17).

Family income

Women living in households that fall within the poorest population quintile use antenatal services much less frequently than do those in the richest 20% (1). Other studies from Kenya show that women in households of high socio-economic status have their first antenatal check 0.17 months earlier than those in households of low socio-economic status(13). Compared with women in the poorest quintile, women in the richest quintile were 4.1 times more likely to initiate timely ANC and 2.6 times more likely to have three or more ANC visits over the course of their pregnancy ($p<0.01$ and $p<0.05$, respectively)(18).

2.3. Needs factors

Pregnancy planned or not

A study on antenatal care service and availability in rural Vietnam shows that if a child had not been planned, i.e. his birth was either mistimed or unwanted; its mother was significantly less likely to initiate timely ANC.

A mother of an unplanned child would be 20 per cent less likely than a mother of a child who wanted to initiate timely ANC and 30 per cent less likely to have three or more ANC visits during that particular pregnancy ($p<0.05$ in both cases)(18).

Younger women, especially teenager, are more likely to have unplanned pregnancies and lack of information and resources to access ANC services (6).

Wantedness of pregnancy

In a study conducted on association between early prenatal care and mother's intention of and desire for the pregnancy, unwanted pregnancy was found to be a predictor of late or no prenatal care. In addition to this, women who were indifferent or did not care about the pregnancy were 3.2 times more likely to obtain late or no prenatal care (7).

Women's attitudes about their pregnancies were associated with inadequate prenatal care, including both inadequate initiation of care and inadequate receipt of services. Women who were unhappy about being pregnant (OR = 1.86), unsure that they wanted to be pregnant (OR = 3.44), or who denied the pregnancy (OR = 6.69) were more likely to have inadequate initiation of care.

Women who were unsure that they wanted to be pregnant (OR = 1.95) or who denied their pregnancies (OR = 2.47) were more likely to have received inadequate care once they had entered care (19). A study done among randomly selected 380 postpartum women on wantedness of pregnancy and prenatal health behaviors in US indicates that women who wanted their pregnancy were more likely to begin prenatal care early (89.8%) than those who did not (65.1%), p < ,001)(20).

Parity

High obstetric risk status was associated with an increased likelihood of late initiation of antenatal care for primiparous women. High obstetric risk primiparous women were 13% more likely to initiate antenatal care after 10 weeks of gestation compared with a low obstetric risk reference group (P= 0.03). Primiparous women considered to be of high obstetric risk and in greatest need for antenatal care were found to be significantly and consistently late in their initiation of the care process (21).

A study on gestational age at antenatal booking in Lagos University Teaching Hospital indicated that nulliparous and primiparous women booked earlier (mean 18.5 ± 8.3 and 18.4 ± 7.4 weeks respectively),than those with parity of 5 , mean 25.9 ± 8.6 weeks and this was statistically significant at (p < 0.0002)(22).

Previous pregnancy experience

Mother's previous pregnancy experience of undesired birth outcome is also one of the positive determinants for maternal health service utilization and early booking (23). In contrast to this, a study done in India revealed that ANC utilization has no association with previous birth outcome (24).

Awareness of care

Awareness of care during pregnancy has positive association with utilization of ANC (25). In study conducted in Ibadan Nigeria, 41.4% of mothers who sought care timely reported that they perceived benefit of the care (26). In another study, reasons for seeking ANC during first trimester by teenagers were reported as wanted pregnancy test and being feeling ill (27).

Perceived quality of service

A study conducted in Harare on the effect of a new antenatal care programme on the attitudes of pregnant women and midwives shows that lack of privacy and insufficient staff at the clinics were a major problem limiting access to antenatal care (28).

Paternal influences

Decision making in the family today in our socio cultural environment is male dominant. In many studies husband's pregnancy intention had a protective effect on the timely initiation of antenatal care. In addition to this pregnancy that were unintended by the mother but were intended by husband had a lower likelihood of delayed care (29-31).

2.4. Conceptual Framework

To conceptualize this study, Andersen and Newman socio-behavioral model framework of health services utilization was used. This framework was first developed in the 1960s and has since gone through four phases. Developed in the 1990s, the framework below represents the fourth phase (5).

According to this model, individual's access to and use of health services is considered to be a function of three characteristics. These are predisposing factors [The socio cultural characteristics of individuals that exist prior to their illness], enabling factors [The logistical aspects of obtaining care] and need factors [The most immediate cause of health service use, from functional and health problems that generate the need for health care services].

Conceptual frame work

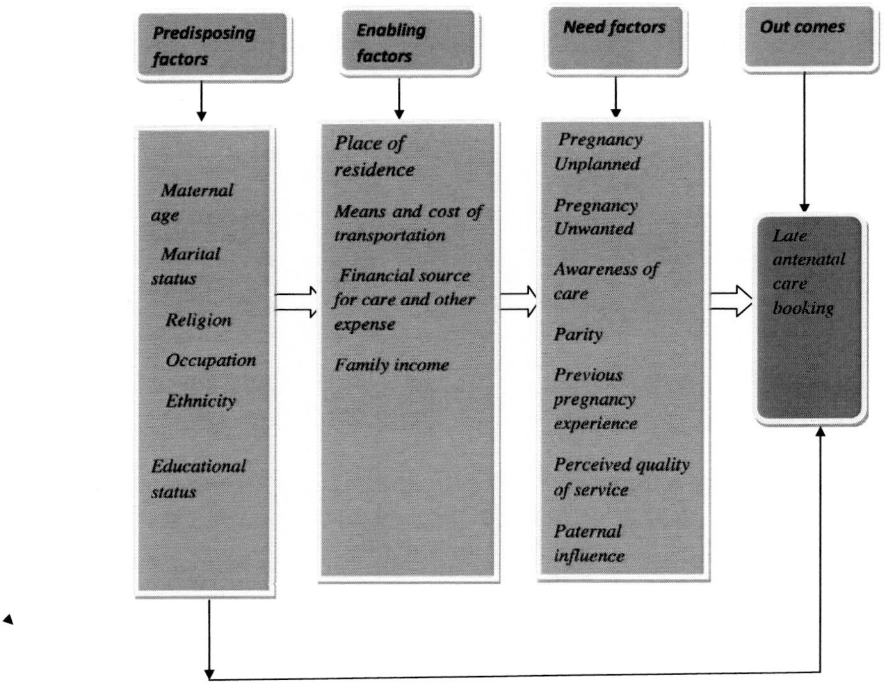

Fig 1.A Conceptual frame work for late antenatal care booking [Adapted from Anderson, 1995] (5)

3. Objectives

3.1 General Objective

1. To determine the magnitude of late antenatal care booking and to identify factors related to the late entry to antenatal care in Gambella Region.

3.2 Specific Objectives

1. To assess the prevalence of late antenatal care booking among pregnant women.

2. To identify factors that predicts late entry to antenatal care in Gambella Region.

3. To assess the knowledge, attitude and practices of pregnant women regarding early initiation of antenatal care.

4. Methodology

4.1. Study Area and period

The study was conducted from March 15 to April 30, 2010 in Gambella Region. The Region has an elevation ranging from 400 to 600 meters above the sea level and largely hot climatic zone. It covers a total area of 23,127sq.km.The capital city of the region is Gambella town which is located at 777km from Addis Ababa, south west of the country. According to the National 2007 census the region has a total population of 306,916. Administratively the region is divided in to three zones and one especial woreda called Ethang. There are about thirteen woredas in the region having different ethnic groups and the regional official working language is Amharic. The majority of ethnic group residing in the region are; Nuer, Agnuhak, and Mezhenger. However, there are also other ethnic groups including settlers from other parts of the country (Oromo, Kembata, Gurage, Tigire, and Amhara) and refuges from the southern Sudan. The region has one hospital, eight health centers, sixty six health post, and seven private clinics (32).

4.2 Study design

Facility based cross-sectional quantitative survey complemented by qualitative method was employed in selected public health facilities of Gambella region.

Quantitative survey: Using structured and pre-tested interviewer-administered questionnaire.

Qualitative Interview: Focus group discussion was used to explore the feeling and beliefs of pregnant women on time of initiation of antenatal care, delay in seeking antenatal care, and other related factors.

4.3 Source and Study population

The source population of the study was all pregnant women in the region during the survey period. The study population of the survey was all pregnant women attending antenatal care in selected public health facilities during the survey period and who are permanent resident of the region.

Inclusion criteria:

- Every pregnant woman visiting the selected public health facilities during the study period and volunteer to respond.
- Pregnant women who are permanent residents (stayed for more than or equal to 6 months) in the study area

Exclusion criteria:

- Participants who were unable to hear, inpatients, unconscious, and mentally disabled.

4.4 Sample size determination

To determine the sample size for the cross-sectional survey design, it was assumed that the precision to an acceptable approximation of the population taking a difference of no more than 5% from the actual figures in the source population and confidence level of 95%. The prevalence of late booking among ANC attendees from previous study was taken to be 76% (5) was used. A non-response rate of 10% considered and then the total sample size was found to be 302. The sample size was calculated using the following formulae:

$$n = \frac{(Z\alpha/2)^2 P (1-p)}{d^2}$$

Where; n=the desired sample size

p=prevalence of late entry to antenatal care among ANC attendees in Addis Ababa (76%) (5)

$Z\alpha/2$= critical value at 95% confidence level of certainty (1.96)

d= the margin of error between the sample and the population =5%

Using the above formula sample size for the single population proportion and considering non response rate of 10%, the total sample size was 302.

For comparing the categories of independent variable with the outcome variable formula for the difference between two proportion was used with the following assumptions: the proportion of unplanned pregnancy in early and late bookers 11.9% and 25.8%(33), type one error of 0.05 and power of 80%, with ratio of early to late bookers is equals to 1 the calculated sample size was 302. Which is the same as the of the single proportion calculations.

4.5 Sampling procedure

The public health facilities which are physically accessible, located in the woredas where majority of the dominant ethnic groups of the region reside, were purposefully selected and included in the study. Accordingly, Gambella hospital, Pugnudo H/C, Abobo H/C, and Metti H/C were included in the study. The sample population for each health facilities was taken by dividing the total sample size in to the respective health facilities proportionate to size of pregnant mothers that were approached and utilized the service in one year before the study based on MCH report from the regional health bureau (34). The pregnant women who attend antenatal care during data collection period were taken consecutively based on the numbers that was set for each health facilities. The procedure continued throughout data collection period until the required sample size was obtained.

4.6. Data collection methods/procedures

Quantitative Study:

The quantitative method of study was conducted by administering structured questionnaire to willing pregnant women. A structured survey questionnaire originally prepared in English was translated in to Amharic and back to English to check for its consistency. Full informed consent was obtained from all eligible participants after explaining the objectives of the study to participants in their own language.

After obtaining informed consent, a local language speaking trained research assistant fluent in Amharic verbally administer questionnaire to respondents. The interview was conducted in private room after they got service in the health facility.

Eight interviewers and four supervisors were employed for data collection. The interviewers were nurses who work in other health facility. They were not appeared with uniform. This was preferred for facilitation of interaction between the respondents and data collection which is important to generate accurate information. Head of MCH unit in the respective data collection sites were used as supervisors for data collectors. The responsibility of data collectors was to fill the questionnaire after obtaining consent from the study participants. The supervisors provide all items necessary for data collection on each data collection day, checking filled questionnaire for completeness and consistency, and solving problems during data collection. Any confusion on data collection procedure was handled by the principal investigator timely.

Qualitative method

Focus Group Discussion was conducted immediately after quantitative data were collected. The principal investigator with one moderator and one note taker carried out one FGD containing 6-8 discussants in each health facility.

4.7. Data quality control

Training: One day training was provided by the principal investigator for data collectors and supervisors on the objective of the research, data collection tools and procedures, how to approach potential respondents and how to keep confidentiality later.

Pretest: Before conducting the main study, pretesting was done in one health center, Gambella town health center, which was later not included in the study. About 5% of the sample was used for pretesting. Final data collection tool was refined based on the findings from the pretesting. All collected data were reviewed and checked for completeness and relevance by the supervisors and principal investigator every day. Data cleaning was done thoroughly by running frequency of variables using Epi/info by the principal investigator before analysis.

4.8. Operational definition

Late antenatal care booking _ includes those pregnant women starting antenatal care after 16 weeks of their pregnancy. This is taken from last menstrual period of the woman.

Predisposing factor- any characteristic of an individual which facilitate or hinder behavior related to health.

Reinforcing factors - are usually societal feedback that encourage or discourage behavior change.

Enabling factors – are usually thought as barriers to behavior changes created by societal factors. Example: limited facilities, lack of income etc.

Booking __ is to mean the first antenatal care visit.

Early antenatal care booking _ includes those pregnant women entering antenatal care before or at16 weeks of gestation.

4.9. Variables in the study

Dependant variable

- ✓ Gestational age at booking

Independent Variables

Predisposing Factors: The socio-cultural/demographic characteristics existing prior to their utilizing service [maternal age, educational status, place of residence, occupation, marital status, ethnicity, religion, parity (primiparae versus multiparae), and attitudes toward the care].

Enabling Factors: This includes the logistical aspects of getting prenatal care [distance from health institution, means and cost of transportation, income, availability and accessibility of health personnel and facilities, and waiting time].

Need Factors: This are factors which contributes for the realization of antenatal care seeking by pregnant women. [Risk awareness i.e. stillbirth, miscarriage or severe congenital anomaly in the past, pregnancy wanted or not, pregnancy planned or not, perceptions on use of early seeking of ANC, any advice from significant others].

Gestational age at which women first presented for antenatal care (Time of initiation of prenatal care) was converted to binary variable. A dichotomous variable was created, with two categories defined as early entry to prenatal care (entry within the first 16 weeks of gestation) and late entry (entry into care later than 16 weeks of gestation). This cut off point was used because it is the common recommendation for developing countries (1).

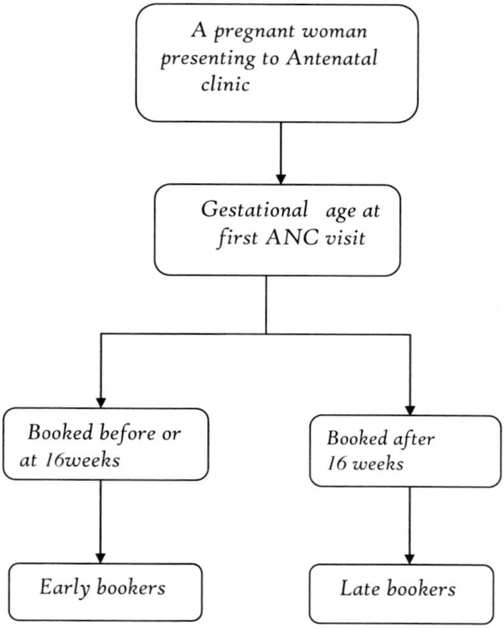

Figure 2: Classification of women according to their booking status among ANC attendees Gambella, April, 2010.

4.10. Statistical data Analysis

First unique code was assigned to each of the completed questionnaire. Then, data entry and cleaning were done by the principal investigator through Epi-info version 3.3.2. Data were exported for analysis to SPSS version 15 statistical package for social sciences software. Descriptive statistics was used, mean and standard deviation for continuous variables and frequency for categorical variables. Analysis was done using bivariate and multivariate logistic regression to observe the effects of independent variables on the outcome variable while simultaneously controlling for other potential confounding factors.

Logistic regression was used to estimate the relative effects of independent variables while adjusting for confounders. Time of entry into prenatal care alone was used to focus on issues that may affect late entry to antenatal care and not issues affecting continuation of prenatal care visits. Since the intent of this study was to focus on entry into prenatal care rather than number of visits.

Those variables that emerged from the bivariate analysis as appearing to be logical and statistically significant predictors of late entry to prenatal care were then used as independent variables in multivariate logistic regression. Variables which showed association in multivariate analysis were considered as final predictors of late entry to prenatal care. The strength of association between different variables and gestational age at booking was measured through odds ratios.

The qualitative part of data were transcribed from a tape recorder and followed by translation from Amharic to English. The summary was coded manually and analyzed by thematic analysis approach.

4.11. Ethical considerations

Ethical clearance was obtained from IRB of Addis Ababa University, Medical faculty. Permission letter to conduct the research was obtained from Gambella regional health bureau for each of the selected health facilities. During data collection, participants were informed about the purpose of the study with their full right to say "*no" (to opt out)*, and it was clearly stated that their decision of "no" by no means affect the service that they obtain from each facilities. The interviewer discussed the issue of confidentiality and request consent before the actual interview was launched. For this purpose, one page consent form was attached as a cover page to each questionnaire. Confidentiality of the information was kept by conducting the interview privately in a single room. In addition, the names of respondents were not included in the questionnaire rather a unique identification number was used. Accordingly, the concern of study subjects for confidentiality was assured.

4.12. Dissemination and utilization of finding

Primarily the final report will be presented to school of public health, AAU. Gambella regional health bureau, interested sectors, and other stakeholders working on reproductive health could also benefit from this research. The extracts of the article will be sent to journals for publication.

5. Result

5.1 Socio demographic characteristics

A total of 302 pregnant women were enrolled in the study giving a response rate of 100%. Of these, 196[64.9%] were in the age group of 15-24, 99 [32.8%] were in the age group of 25-34, and the rest 7[2.3%] were in the age group of greater than or equal to 35years. The mean age (±SD) of the respondents was found to be 23±4.83, ranging from 15-47years.

The ethnic composition of the respondents were Agnuak, Nuer, Mejengir, and followed by others high landers 109[36.1%], 46[15.2%], 52[17.2%], and 95[31.5%] respectively. In regard to their religion respondents of Protestant were found to be 223[73.8%], followed by Orthodox 46[15.2%], Muslim 23[7.6%], and others 10[3.3%]. Two hundred seventy three were married or in union. One hundred fifty had primary education while, two hundred two were unemployed. One hundred eighty-eight (62.3%), of the respondents did not pay for transportation during their visit to the health facilities while the rest paid less than or equal to 10 Eth birr. Thirty eight percent used taxi service as means of transportation to access the health facility, the cost of which range from 2-10 Eth. birr depending on the proximity to the health facility.

Table 1 Socio- demographic characteristics of respondents, Gambella, South west of Ethiopia April, 2010.

Variables	Number	Percent
Age in years (N=302)		
15- 24	196	64.9
25-34	99	32.8
≥35	7	2.3
Mean ± SD	23±4.83 yrs	
Ethnicity (N=302)		
Agnuak	109	36.1
Nuer	46	15.2
Mejengir	52	17.2
Others	95	31.5
Residential area(N=302)		
Urban	151	50
Rural	151	50
Religion(N=302)		
Protestant	223	73.8
Orthodox	46	15.2
Muslim	23	7.6
Others**	10	3.3
Marital status(N=302)		
Married	273	90.4
Single/never married	7	2.3
Separated/Divorced or Widowed	22	7.3
Educational status(N=302)		
Illiterate	93	30.8
Elementary/Grade 1-8	150	49.7
High school/Grade 9-12	47	15.6
Diploma and above	12	4
Average family income/month(ETB) (N=302)		
≤ 300 Eth. birr	92	30.5
301-500 Eth. birr	50	16.6
501-1000 Eth. birr	91	30.1
≥ 1001 Eth. birr	69	22.8
Cost of transportation		
No cost paid	188	62.3
≤10 Eth. birr	144	37.7

*** Includes Catholic, Wakefeta and no religion*

5.2. Pregnancy duration at entry to ANC

A large number of women entered ANC late 145[48%], and the proportion of respondents who made their visit with in the recommended period of time [before or at 16 weeks] was found to be 157[52%]. The mean pregnancy duration (±SD) at entry to ANC was 4.6±1.4 month ranging from 1month to 9 months.

5.3. Past and present obstetric history

Two hundred six, [68.2%], were multiparous while the rest 96[31.8%] were nulliparous women. Two hundred eighty of respondents had no history of previous abortion while the rest 22 had a history of at least one abortion. One hundred seventy seven of the respondents had less than three children and twenty had four and above children. Twenty respondents had history of death of one child, five had history of death of two and above child, and six respondents had at least one history of stillbirth. Most of the respondents, 273[90.4%] had no problem in the last delivery while, 29[9.6%] had a problem in the last delivery. Only twelve of the respondents had a history of previous caesarean delivery.

Table2. Obstetrics history of respondents cross tabulated by gestational age at booking among ANC attendees, Gambella, April, 2010

Variables	Gestational age at booking		Total
	Booked timely (≤16weeks) No[%]	Booked late (>16weeks) No[%]	
Parity			
Nulliparous	50[52.1]	46[47.9]	96[100]
Para≥1	107[51.9]	99[48.1]	206[100]
History of abortion			
Yes	12[54.5]	10[45.5]	22[100]
No	145[51.8]	135[48.2]	280[100]
Number of children(n=197)			
<3children	91[51.4]	86[48.6]	177[100]
≥3children	11[55]	9[45]	20[100]
No of children died(n=25)			
1 child died	12[60]	8[40]	20[100]
≥2 child died	0[0.00%]	5[100]	5[100]
Problem in the last delivery			
Yes	15[51.7]	14[48.3]	29[100]
No	142[52]	131[48]	273[100]
Previous caesarean delivery			
Yes	5[41.7]	7[58.3]	12[100]
No	152[52.4]	138[47.6]	290[100]

5.4. Knowledge of Antenatal care

Two hundred ninety one [96.4%] of the respondents perceived as ANC is highly important for the health of the mother while the rest, 11[3.6%] perceived and rated as medium for the health of the mother. Majority, 273[90.4%] of the respondents perceived and rated ANC as highly important for the health of the fetus while, 29[9.6%] as medium or less important.

When asked the best time in pregnancy to begin antenatal care, in figure (35%) stated that the first trimester was ideal. However, each of the women went on describing a range of barriers that made early booking difficult.

5.5. History of service utilization

Most of the women suspected pregnancy when they first missed their period. Some of the women waited until two or three missed periods before concluding that they were pregnant. The parous women also recognized familiar signs of pregnancy. Pregnancy confirmation was one of the reasons for the first visit to the health facilities. Two hundred fifty five (74.5%) of respondents were in their second trimester, 55(18.2%) were in their first trimester, and the rest 22(7.3%) in their third trimester of pregnancies when they first visit health facilities (Fig3 below).

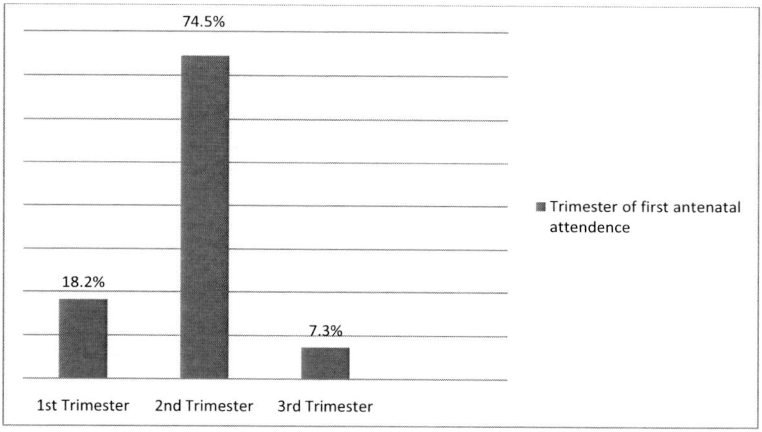

Fig3 Trimester of first antenatal clinic attendance among ANC attendees in Gambella, April, 2010

One hundred twenty-seven of the respondents had no history of previous ANC attendance while the rest one hundred seventy five had ever attendance of antenatal care. Of one hundred seventy five respondents who respond to the timing of first antenatal care visit for the pregnancy preceding the current pregnancy one hundred ten had made their first visit before or at 16weeks of their gestation while the rest sixty five had made their first ANC visit after 16weeks of gestation.

Table3 Past utilization of ANC by gestational age at booking of respondents, Gambella, April, 2010

Variables		Gestational age at booking		
		Booked timely No[%]	Booked Late No[%]	Total No[%]
Ever attendance of ANC	Yes	93[53.1]	82[46.9]	175[100]
	No	64[50.4]	63[49.6]	127[100]
ANC experience of preceding pregnancy	Booked ≤16 weeks	75[68.2]	35[31.8]	110[100]
	Booked >16weeks	18[27.7]	47[72.3]	65[100]
Perceived number of ANC visits	< 4 visits	83[100]	83[100]	166[100]
	≥ 4 visits	74[54.4]	62[45.6]	136[100]

Regarding the payment for the service, 110[62.85%] had not paid for the service that they utilized while, 65[37.14%] paid for the service they utilized. The reason for the payment was, 20[30.77%] for consultation, 55[84.64%] for laboratory, 9[13.84%] for ultrasound and the rest 8[12.30%] paid for drugs. Thirty-nine [60%] paid less than or equal to10 Eth. birr, and the rest 26[40%] paid greater than 10 Eth. birr.

Table 4 Satisfaction status of respondents towards staff approach, laboratory, waiting time and privacy among pregnant mothers attending ANC in Gambella, April, 2010

Variables	Number	Percent
Staff approach :n=175		
Highly satisfied	128	73.10
Satisfied	47	26.90
Laboratory :n=175		
Highly satisfied	113	64.6
Satisfied	54	30.9
Medium /Not satisfied/highly unsatisfied	8	4.6
Waiting time :n=175		
Highly satisfied	111	63.4
Satisfied	54	30.9
Medium /Not satisfied	10	5.7
Privacy :n=175		
Highly satisfied	124	70.9
Satisfied /Medium /Not satisfied	51	29.1

5.6. History of current pregnancy and ANC

Twenty eight [9.3%], of the respondents knew that they were pregnant when they missed menses once, 98 [32.5%] missed a period twice, 135[44.7%] missed a period three times and above, while the rest knew through laboratory examination/urine test 70[23.2%], 74[24.5%] through physiological changes and sign and symptoms that they observed on them.

Two hundred-nine [69.2%] of the respondents reported that their current pregnancy was planned while, 93[30.8%] reported that their current pregnancy was unplanned. In almost all, [99.7%], of the respondents having planned pregnancy the plan was made with their husbands.

Among the 93 unplanned pregnancy, 57[61.3%] were wanted by the mother, 36 [38.7%] were not wanted by the mother, 48[51.6%] were wanted by their husbands, and 45[48.3%] were not wanted by their husbands after the conception.

Thirty-three [10.9%] of the respondents faced pregnancy related problems in the current pregnancy. About 143[47.3%] of the respondents reported that they got an advice to come and attend ANC. The sources of advices were community health workers 71[49.7%], husband 51 [35.7%], mother or sister 16[11.2%], and others 5[3.5%]. One hundred fifty-seven [52%] of the respondents made their first visit before 4months and the rest 145[48. %] registered after 4months of gestation.

5.7 Reason for booking at the time of entry

Respondents were asked why they prefer that specific time to initiate antenatal care. The reason for registering/booking at the time of entry to prenatal care reported by the respondents was that they thought it was appropriate time, booking at convenient time, time constraints, financial constraints and others.

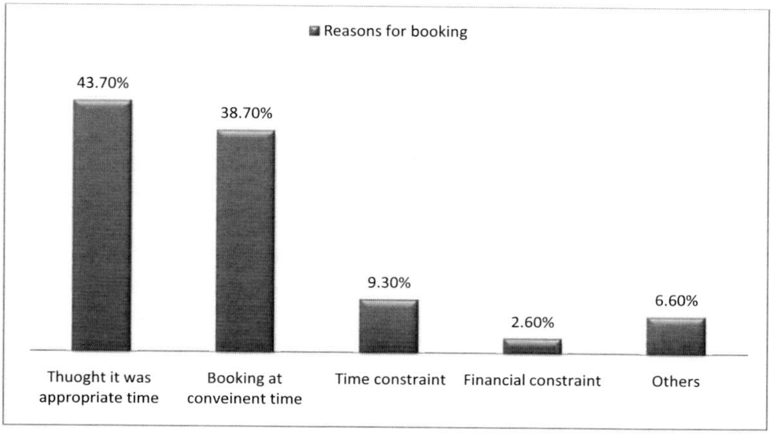

Figure4. Reason for booking at the time of entry to prenatal care among pregnant women, Gambella, April, 2010

5.8 Factors affecting late entry to antenatal care

Significance levels of variables were determined using bivariate and multivariate logistic regression models. Time of entry to prenatal care was compared on key socio demographic variables, obstetric history variables, knowledge of ANC, previous service utilization, history of current pregnancy and reasons for booking at the time of entry to antenatal care.

Bivariate analysis showed that respondents who had unplanned pregnancy, who perceived that the appropriate time to register for antenatal care was after 16weeks of gestation, who were booked after 16weeks for the pregnancy preceding the current pregnancy, and those whose reason for booking at the time of entry to prenatal care was thought it was delay due to time constraint and appropriate time for booking were more likely to initiate prenatal care late than others[OR=1.68,95%CI[1.03,2.79]],[OR=1.79,95%CI[1.11,2.900]],[OR=1.82,95%CI[1.37,2.44]],[OR=10.5,95%[3.15,36.24]],[OR=2.61,95%CI[1.625,4.2]],respectively.(Table 5)

Whereas, other variables like socio demographic, parity of mother, knowledge of antenatal care, problem in the last delivery, previous caesarean delivery, wantedness of pregnancy, and problem in the index pregnancy were found to have no significant relationship with gestational age at booking in the bivariate analysis.

In a multivariate logistic regression, three factors were found to be statistically associated with late entry to antenatal care booking after adjusting for other variables. Women who had unplanned pregnancy were 2.85 times more likely to enter prenatal care late compared to women having planned pregnancy [OR=2.85, 95%CI [1.274, 6.355]]. Women who had booked after 16 weeks of gestation for the pregnancy preceding the current pregnancy were 5.85 times more likely to enter prenatal care late [OR=5.85, 95%CI [2.665 12.828]] compared to others. Those women whose reason for their booking at the time of entry to prenatal care was thought it was appropriate time for booking were found to be 2.15 times more likely to book late when compared to others [OR=2.15, 95%CI [1.052,4.379]].[Table 5 below]

Table5. Factors influencing late entry to antenatal care among pregnant women attending ANC, Gambella, 2010

Variables		***Gestational age at booking***		***COR [95% CI]***	***AOR [95% CI]***
		Booked Late No[%]	**Booked timely No[%]**		
Pregnancy Planned	Yes	92[63.4]	117[74.5]	1.00	1.00
	No	53[36.6]	40[25.5]	1.685[1.03,2.76]**	**2.846[1.274,6.355]**
Perception on appt. time of booking(weeks)	Perceived ≤ 16	41[28.3]	65[41.1]	1.00	1.00
	Perceived > 16	104[71.7]	92[58.6]	1.792[1.108,2.9]**	1.41[0.627,3.167]
Past experience of timing(wks)	Booked ≤ 16	35[42.7]	75[80.6]	1.00	1.00
	Booked > 16	47[57.3]	18[19.4]	1.823[1.37,2.44]**	**5.85[2.665,12.828]**
Reason for booking was told the time was appropriate for them	Yes	46[34.8%]	86[65.2%]	1.00	1.00
	No	99[58.2%]	71[41.8%]	2.61[1.625,4.2]**	**2.147[1.052,4.379]**
Parity	Para≥1	99[48.1%]	107[51.9%]	1.00	1.00
	Para = 0	46[47.9%]	50[52.1%]	0.994[0.612,1.62]	0.94[0.612,1.6125]

5.9 Result from qualitative study

To support the finding from the quantitative data, four focus groups discussions were conducted. Participants were volunteer pregnant mothers attending antenatal care in those selected public health facilities during the survey. Two focus group discussions were conducted among women who initiated antenatal care early within 16th weeks of gestation (n=8 participants /each) and the rest two focus groups (n=6 & 7 participants each) discussions were conducted with late initiators of antenatal care.

Before the discussion is started, the process was fully explained to the participants with a view to obtain their informed consent. Voluntary participation was emphasized, and the participants were given a chance to ask questions. They were assured of confidentiality of the information provided. Their permission was sought first before the interview was tape-recorded. They were informed that they were free to withdraw from the study at any time if they so wished and that their withdrawal would not affect their antenatal care in any way.

Eligibility to either group was obtained through giving information that addressed when they first received prenatal care and when they first realized/confirmed their pregnancy. This information was used to group participants into categories of late and early initiators of antenatal care. The focus group discussions were recorded and transcribed verbatim and data were organized by session with no personal identifiers.

The focus groups discussions were conducted with the discussant based on the following thematic areas of discussions:

1. Attitude towards pregnancy
2. Pregnancy symptoms knowledge
3. Social Support
4. Timelines of clinic visit.

Early initiators were more knowledgeable of pregnancy signs and symptoms, whereas late initiators seemed to be unaware of signs and symptoms. Younger participants, particularly, seemed less aware of the signs and symptoms of pregnancy.

The early and late group participants all had a clear picture of the importance of prenatal care and the positive effects it can have on the mother's and child's health.

Majority of women participating in the focus group discussions agreed that prenatal care was important but maybe not to their current pregnancy, especially among late initiators. All the women could give several reasons on why to seek prenatal care, but often expressed their beliefs that even if they sought prenatal care, there was still a chance that there could be pregnancy complications.

The following statements are the voices of the study participants addressing some of the domains and common themes identified in the study.

5.10 Attitude towards pregnancy

Early initiators

The early initiators of prenatal care had a positive attitude towards their being pregnant. Most of the discussants who initiated the care timely informed their getting pregnant to their husbands. One of the discussant who initiated antenatal care at 4th months of her gestation claimed that

"I knew that I was pregnant when I missed a period/menses...

I was happy with my getting pregnant and so was my husband."

On the other hand late initiators of antenatal care seemed to have less inclination towards their getting pregnant.

Some of the early bookers come to health facility so as to confirm their pregnancy via laboratory examination. A woman claimed that she started booking at first month of her pregnancy, because she faced abortion for the pregnancy preceding the current pregnancy.

"I started this check up in the first month soon I missed my period.

I had had abortion before.

I started this check up early because I fear the past happenings".

Late initiators

Some of the respondents mentioned that it was important to book early in pregnancy in order to get care later in the labour, as one who booked at 6months, explained.

> *"It is good to go to the clinic because when you are in labour...*
>
> *They ask first whether you had attended antenatal care or not and your card....*
>
> *They give an emphasis and priority for those who had a card and attended antenatal care..."*

This was the reported experience of one of the older woman, who had not booked on her previous pregnancy and she decided to book at this time because of it.

5.11 Pregnancy Symptoms Knowledge

Early initiators

Most women who had previous pregnancies described signs of pregnancy that they recognized; one of the discussant explained that:

> *"I just felt life inside me ...*
>
> *My breast was getting bigger...*
>
> *The nipple around it started to get black."*

Early initiators seemed to have more knowhow about the signs of pregnancy. One of the respondent responded as:

"I knew I was a pregnant when I missed period....

Once I found out I was pregnant, and I was like Okay...

Time to go and attend prenatal care monthly"

Late initiators

On the other hand, late initiators and those with no previous pregnancy experience demonstrated relatively less knowledge about the signs of pregnancy and they were unsure of getting pregnant. One of the discussant who booked after 4months responded as:

"This is my first time pregnancy...

I was not sure that I was pregnant...

I had been using Depo provera and had amenorrhea."

5.12 Social Support

Early initiators

Most of the early initiators had a strong support from significant others when compared to that of late initiators of prenatal care. Woman who booked within the recommended period of booking claimed that:

"I get a support from my husband...

I don't prepare food or wash my clothes...

Somebody do that for me."

Late initiators

In contrast with that of early initiators of prenatal care those discussants that started their first antenatal care visit after 16th weeks of their gestation had, comparably, less social support during their pregnancy.

> *"I don't have any person who takes care of me during my pregnancy...*
>
> *My husband is not living with me...*
>
> *There is no one who remind me the date of appointment for the prenatal care follow up."*

5.13 Timelines of clinic visit

Early initiators

Early initiators of focus groups discussions initiated the care within the recommended period of time because they had positive attitude towards their being pregnant, have strong social support, and seemed to be more knowledgeable about the symptoms of pregnancy than that of late initiators of prenatal care. One of the discussant who booked with in the first 4th months responded as:

"I informed to my husband that I get pregnant. He said ok, and happy with my getting pregnant. Because I knew that the appropriate time to book for antenatal care is within the first four months of gestation I come to health facility and started the follow up".

Late initiators

When compared with early initiators of prenatal care, late initiators of prenatal care were failing to book within the recommended period of time due to several reasons. Some of this reasons which favors late booking were unawareness of service, unavailability of the service and residential area. One of the discussant who booked at 7th months of here gestation responded that:

"My very reason to seek prenatal care at 7th months...

I live in the rural area of Gambella called 'Abol'....

The area was far and remote where I can't find any health facility....

I have to cover a long distance on my foot....

So that l can get health facility and attend prenatal care."

Some participants commented that it is appropriate to begin antenatal care only once the fetus can be felt moving. Mother who booked at 6months at Gog health center stated that:

"You can't just go to the health facility without feeling the baby moving....

In case they ask you at the clinic what do you feel?

If you don't feel anything, what do you say?"

Table5. Summary response of focus group discussant regarding antenatal care, Gambella, 2010

Variable	Antenatal care importance	Attitude towards pregnancy	Timelines of ANC visit	Social support
Early initiators	Important	Excited, jubilant	prompt	strong support
Late initiators	Important	Disinterested	delayed visit	less social support

As indicated above early initiators of prenatal care were excited about becoming pregnant. This response contracts with that of late initiators who were disinterested of becoming a pregnant.

6. Discussion

The study attempted to assess the proportion of women who entered antenatal care late in Gambella, South west Ethiopia, in 2010 and identified related factors.

One hundred forty five [48%] of respondents entered prenatal care late in their pregnancies. The time of first entry to prenatal care ranges from 1st month of last menstrual period to 9th months of gestation. The proportion of women who entered to prenatal care after 16weeks of gestation in the current study was higher than that of the New South Wales, Australia [41%], but smaller than the findings of the studies conducted in South Western Nigeria[82.6%.], Addis Ababa [59.8], and EDHS 2005[94%] (3, 4, 6, 26).

The mean gestational age at booking for all pregnant women was 4.6 months which was in comparable with the findings from the studies conducted in Nigeria, and Addis Ababa, Ethiopia (9, 26, 33). However it was lower than 6 months reported amongst pregnant women in Enugu, south east of Nigeria(35).

The booking pattern was found not to be influenced by socio-demographic factors. In accordance with the finding from EDHS 2005, maternal education was not seen as statistically significant factor for late entry to prenatal care in this study(3). However, in contrast to other studies the present study did not find out statistically significant association between maternal age, marital status, and occupation and time of entry to prenatal care (6-15).

Parity of women was found to be statistically associated with gestational age at booking in studies done in England and Enugu, south west of Nigeria(21, 35).

This study, however, did not replicate that finding. A statistically significant association was not found between parity of the mother and time of entry to prenatal care.

Previous obstetric complications such as still birth and caesarean section have no influence on gestational age at booking which were also reported in study conducted in Nigeria(26). This might be due to the negative effect of ignorance which had been demonstrated in vicious circle of disease, ignorance and poverty. On the other hand, information collected from focus group discussions suggested that undesired birth outcome experiences were seen as a factor for early entry to prenatal care. The finding from focus group discussion is similar with that of study done in Bangladesh(23).

Earlier awareness and less ambivalence could be more likely among women who are consciously planning to become pregnant and thus watching for relevant signs. Women who are initially ambivalent about being pregnant may be more likely to deny early signs and to delay confirming pregnancy or seeking care. Multivariate analysis indicated that those respondents having unplanned pregnancy were 2.85 times more likely to enter prenatal care late when compared to those who planned their pregnancies. This might be due to the fact that those women who did not plan their pregnancies were not well prepared physically, financially, and emotionally to deal with pregnancy. This finding was in line with the finding of the studies done in Vietnam and New South Wales, Australia (6, 18).

The study of Kupek et al (2002) looking at predictive factors of late initiation of antenatal care in England and Wales also found that unplanned pregnancy was associated with late booking of antenatal care (21).

However, even if majority of unplanned pregnancies were wanted, wantedness of the pregnancy did not show statistically significant association with time of entry to prenatal care. This finding was not in accordance with the findings of the studies done in Missouri, England and Nigeria (7, 19-22).

Both groups of respondents who entered prenatal care late and those entered with in recommended period of time agreed that prenatal care was important both for the health of the mothers and the fetus. This finding was supported by finding from focus group discussion of pregnant mothers.

Sixty five percent of respondents perceived that the appropriate time to register for antenatal care was after 16 weeks of their gestation. Respondents who perceived that the appropriate time to register for antenatal care was after 16weeks of gestation were 1.85 times more likely to enter prenatal care late compared to others.

Finding of this study was in agreement with the study conducted in Addis Ababa(33) on time of entry to ANC for the pregnancy preceding the current pregnancy and late booking. In multivariate analysis respondents who failed to initiate prenatal care with in the first 16weeks of gestation for the pregnancy preceding the current pregnancy were found 5.85 times more likely to enter prenatal care late when compared to those who initiated prenatal care within the recommended period.

Illness in index pregnancy that was found to be significantly associated with late booking in other study had no influence on gestational age at booking in this study(29). However, in agreement with current study another study from south west Nigeria showed no association between illness in index pregnancy and late entry to antenatal care.

This might be due to poor counseling of those who had illness in the index pregnancy by the health workers that they first had contact with.

Traditionally, nulliparous women would first seek counseling from multiparous women who were considered to be more experienced and would eventually in most instances discourage early booking(9).

Respondents had several reasons for booking at the time of entry to prenatal care. The major reason for booking at the gestational age that they thought was it was the appropriate time to initiate antenatal care. Respondents whose reason for booking at the time of entry to prenatal care was that they thought it was appropriate time to initiate antenatal care were more likely to initiate prenatal care late than others. This might be due to lack of appropriate information on antenatal care.

In bivariate analysis, respondents whose reason for entry to prenatal care at the time of gestational booking was due to time constraint were 10.5 times more likely to initiate antenatal care late when compared to others. This finding was supported by the finding from the qualitative part of the study.

Previous caesarean delivery and abortion for the pregnancy preceding the current pregnancies that were found to have statistically significant association with time of booking in the study done in New South Wales, Australia (6) had an influence on time of entry to prenatal care as envisaged in the qualitative aspect of this study. This might be due to the reason that women who have had a previous caesarean delivery are aware of the risk of pregnancy complications and therefore more likely to seek ANC early.

7. Strength and Limitation of the study

7.1 Strength of the study

The study used focus groups discussions to strengthen the findings from quantitative study. Multiple logistic regressions were also employed to control for potential confounding factors. The study was conducted in Gambella region, where research findings are deficient to make evidence based decision for program implementation.

7.2. Limitation of the study

This study has considered pregnant women attending ANC in the selected governmental health institutions during the study period. Governmental health facilities are preferred because it is the first contact and easily accessible to the community for preventive health care aspects. Despite these assumptions, other pregnant women may visit private clinics and hospitals for ANC. There could be some socio-demographic differences as those pregnant mothers visiting other health institutions. This study is limited to address pregnant women those attended ANC other than the public health centers. In addition to this the public health facilities which are physically accessible, and located in the woreda where the majority of the ethnic groups reside were purposefully selected and included in the study. Furthermore, as the interviewers used were nurses, who were different from service provider, not appeared with uniform, the participants can identify them and their might be probability of social desirability bias.

8. Conclusion

- Importance of antenatal care both for the health of the mother and the fetus was recognized by large majority of respondents.
- Late entry to antenatal care still remains relatively high in the study area indicating that the importance of early booking is yet to be promoted.
- Unplanned pregnancy was found to be a significant predictor of failure to initiate prenatal care with in the first 16weeks of gestational age amongst pregnant women.
- Untimely entry to prenatal care for the pregnancy preceding the current pregnancy was associated with late booking.
- Undesired birth outcome experiences were found to be a factor for early entry for antenatal care as envisaged in the qualitative aspect of the study.
- The major reason for entry to prenatal care at the time of booking was that they thought that the time was appropriate for their booking.

9. Recommendation

- There is need for public enlightenment and incorporation of the benefits of early booking in the routine antenatal health education.
- Attention should be directed toward women's perceived reasons for not initiating early care.
- There is a need for further research to identify the specific concerns of late bookers and areas where new intervention might encourage the uptake of the service.
- Future community based studies should include other potential factors and expand to other aspects of ANC such as number of ANC visits, services provided during ANC visits and satisfaction of women and providers.
- The FMOH should develop a clear guideline on maternal antenatal care which includes detailed protocols for urgent booking of women presenting late.

10. References

1. *Carla A, Blanc A, Van P. ANC in developing countries, promises, achievements and missed opportunities; an analysis of trends, levels and differentials, 1990-2001. Geneva2003.*
2. *WHO. Antenatal Care. Report of a Technical Working Group 1994 - WHO/FRH/MSM/968 1994.*
3. *CSA. Central statistical Authority and ORC Macro. Addis Ababa 2005.*
4. *Fantahun M. Factors Affecting ANC attendance and preference of place of Delivery by pregnant women in Gulele district Addis Ababa: Addis Ababa University; 2000.*
5. *Andersen R. Revisiting the behaviuoral model and access to medical care:does it matter? Journal of health and social behaviour 1995;36:1-10.*
6. *Lieu T, Rubin G. Late entry to antenatal care in New South Wales, Australia. Reproductive Health journal 2006;3(8).*
7. *Hulsey TM. Association between early prenatal care and mother's intention and desire for the Pregnancy. JOGNN 2001;30(3).*
8. *Raatikainen K, Heiskanen N, Heinonen S. Under-attending free antenatal care is associated with adverse pregnancy outcomes. BMC Public Health 2007;7(268).*
9. *Adekanle DA, Isawumi A. Late antenatal care booking and its predictors among pregnant women in South Western Nigeria. Online Journal of Health and Allied Sciences 2008; 7(1).*
10. *Mekonnen Y, Mekonnen A. Factors influencing the use of maternal healthcare services in Ethiopia. Journal of Health and Population Nutrition 2003;21(4):374-82.*
11. *Al-Shammari SA, Khoja T, Jarallah JS. The pattern of antenatal visits with emphasis on gestational age at booking in Riyadh health centres. Journal of the Royal Society for the promotion of Health 1994; 114(2): 62-6.*
12. *Isaranurug S, Chompikul J, Erlindawati. Factors related to the utilization of antenatal care service among pregnant women at health centers in Aceh Besar district,Nanggroe Aceh Darussalam province, Indonesia. Journal of Public Health and Development 2008;6 (2).*

13. *Magadi MA, Madise NJ, Rodrigues RN. Frequency and timing of antenatal care in Kenya: explaining the variations between women of different communities. Social Science & Medicine 2000; 51(4): 551-61.*
14. *Pagnini DL, Reichman NE. Psychosocial factors and the timing of prenatal care among women in New Jersey's HealthStart Program. Family Planning Perspectives2000; 32(2): 56–64.*
15. *Jewkes R, Abrahams N, Mvo Z, Rowe R, Garcia J. Social class, ethnicity and attendance for antenatal care in the United Kingdom: a systematic review. Journal of Public Health Medicine 2003;25(2): 113-9.*
16. *Alderliesten M, Vrijkotte T, Van der wal M, Bonsel G. Late start of antenatal care among ethnic minorities in a large cohort of pregnant women. British Journal of Obstetrics and Gynecology 2007;114:1232-9.*
17. *Mekonnen Y. pattern of maternal health service utilization in Southern Ethiopia. Evidence from community and family survey. EthiopJHealth Dev 2003;17(1):27-33.*
18. *Do M. Antenatal care service availability and utilization in rural Viet Nam. Asia-Pacific Population Journal 2008;23 (1):30-54.*
19. *Marjorie R. Sable, Wilkinson DS. pregnancy intentions, pregnancy attitudes, and the use of prenatal care in Missouri. Maternal and child health journal 1998; 2(3).*
20. *Altfeld S, Handler A, Burton D, Berman L. Wantedness of pregnancy and prenatal health behaviors. Women & Health1998;26(4):29-43.*
21. *Kupek E, Petrou S, Vause S, Maresh M. Clinical, provider and socio demographic predictors of late initiation of antenatal care in England and Wale. International Journal of Obstetrics and Gynaecology 2002 109(7):265-73*
22. *Adegbola O. Gestational age at antenatal booking in Lagos University Teaching Hospital . Nig Q J Hosp Med 2008; 18(2): 79-82.*
23. *Chakrborty N, Islam A, Barri W. Determinants of the use of maternal health service in rural Bangladish. Health promotion International 2003; 18(4):327.*
24. *Champman R. Endangering safe motherhood in Mozambique. ANC as pregnancy risk. Social Science and Medicine 2003;57(1).*
25. *Chandiok N, Dhillon B , Kambo I. Determinanats of ANC utilization in rural areas of India Journal of Obstetric and Gynecology India 2006;56(1):47-52.*

26. *Okunlola M, Ayinde O, Owonikoko K. Factors influencing gestational age at ANC booking at the university college hospital, Ibadan, Nigeria Journal of Obstetrics and Gynecology 2006;26(3):195-7.*
27. *Lee SH. Pregnant teenagers' reasons for seeking or delaying ANC Clinical nurse Reserch1999;4(1):38-49.*
28. *Murira N, Munjanj SP, Zhanda I, Nystrom L, Lindmark G. Effect of a new antenatal care programme on the attitudes of pregnant women and midwives towards antenatal care in Harare. Central African Journal of Medicine1997 43(5):131-5*
29. *Gharoro EP, Igbafe A. Antenatal care some characteristics of the booking visit in a major teaching hospital in the developing world Medical Science Monitoring 2000; 6(3):519-22.*
30. *Rowe Re, Magee H, Quigley MA, Heron P, Askham J, Brocklehurst P. Social and ethnic differences in attendance for antenatal care in England. Public Health 2008;122(12):1363-72.*
31. *Sangi-Haghpeykar H, Mehta M, Posner S, Poindexter A. Paternal influences on the timing of prenatal pare among hispanics. Maternal and Child Health Journal 2005;9(2).*
32. *FDRE. Summary and statistical report of the 2007 population and housing census Addis Ababa, Ethiopia 2008.*
33. *Tariku A. Why pregnant women delay to attend prenatal care? cross sectional study on timing of first antenatal care at public health institution Addis Ababa: Addis Ababa University; 2007.*
34. *RHB. Gambella Regional Health Bureau annual report. Gambella 2001*
35. *Nwagha. UI, UGgwu OV, Nwagha T, Anyaehie US. The influence of parity on gestational age at booking among pregnant women in Enugu,South East Nigeria Nigerian Journal of Physiological Sciences 2008; 23(1-2):67 - 70.*

Annexes

Annex I. sampling procedure

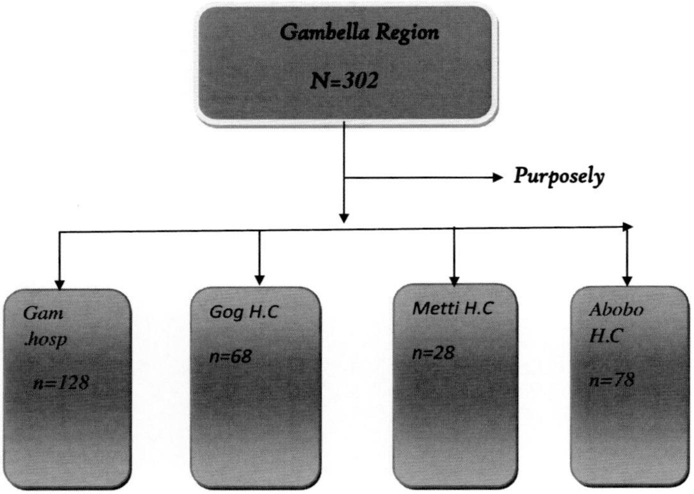

Fig4. Schematic presentation of sampling procedure, Gambella, 2010

Annex II Informed Consent Sheet

I Study Information sheet

Good morning /afternoon, my name is_________________________ and I am a midwife/nurse working for this hospital/health center. I am also a part of a team carrying out study on late antenatal care booking and its predictors among pregnant women attending antenatal care in the region. Currently, we are conducting a study on late antenatal care booking and factors contributing for delay in initiation of antenatal care. The purpose of this study is to identify possible factors contributing to late antenatal care booking and its predictors among pregnant women. There will not be any an immediate benefit in terms of money; rather you may be morally satisfied for you contribute to the community welfare that may be attained from the result of the study. We believe that the study findings will help in order to improve care for mothers and their newborns.

If you participate in the study, it will not take us more than 15 minutes. Your name will not be written on this form, thus the information you provide will not be known to others. There is no risk involved in participating in the study. Your participation is purely voluntary, and you can withdraw any time after you get involved in the study without compromising the services you ought to get from the hospital/health center. However, we hope that you will participate in this study since your views are important.

Do you have any questions?

If you have any question you can contact the principal investigator at any time convenient for you using the following address:

Name of principal Investigator- Tariku Endeshaw Alemu

Address- Addis Ababa University, School of public health

Addis Ababa, Ethiopia

Cell phone 0912082134

E-mail endashawtariku@yahoo.com

Addis Ababa University, Medical Faculty, IRB

Phone No 011553873

E- Mail aaumfirb@yahoo.com

II. Consent form

I, the selected participant, heard the information in the consent sheet and understood what is required from me and what will happen to me if I take part in the study. I understand that all the information regarding me, like name and all answers given by me must not be transferred to the third party. I can also understand that I can withdraw from the study at any time without giving a reason and without me or my families' routine service utilization being affected for my refusal.

Now please tell me if you agree to participate in the interview.

The Participant:

1. Agreed ☐

2. Did not agree ☐ → End the interview and thank the respondent.

Interviewer Agreement

I certify that I have taken written consent from the respondent that she has agreed to participate in study and I have confirmed the agreement is correct.

Interviewer Name: ______________________ Signature______________________

|____________|__________| 2010.

Date month

Supervisor Name: ______________________ Signature______________________

|____________|__________| 2010.

Date month

Addis Ababa University, Medical Faculty IRB

Phone No 0115538734

E-Mail aaumfirb@yahoo.com

Structured Questionnaires

Mother's code...... |_______|_______|_______|	Date |_______|_______| 2010		
Interviewer's Name________________	Interviewer's code .... |_______|_______|		
Start Time _____:____	End time_____:_______		

Number	Question	Response	Skip	Code

Section I Socio-demographic variables

1.	Age	____years		
2.	Ethnic	1. Nuer 2. Agnuhak 3. Mejengir 4 Amhara 5. Oromo 6.Others [Specify]___________		
3.	Residential area	1. Urban______ 2. Rural_______		
4.	Religion	1. Orthodox 2. Protestant 3. Muslim 4. Catholic 5. Others [Specify]___________		
5.	What is your current marital status?	1. Single /Never married 2. Married/Living together 3. Divorced/Separated 4. Widowed		
6.	Did you ever attend a school?	1. Yes 2. No→	8.	

7.	What was the highest grade you completed?	1. Grades ______ 2. Tech/voc. Certificate 3. University/College Diploma 4. University/College Degree 5. Don't Know.		
8.	What is your occupation?	1. Government employee 2. Private sector employee 3. Self employed 4. Housewife 5. Farmer 6. Others[Specify]__________		
9.	How much is your average family income per month.	Monthly income________ Eth birr		
10	Cost of transportation paid for coming to health facility and back to home.	1. No cost paid at all 2. _______Eth birr		

Section II obstetrics History

11	How many times have you been pregnant?	1. ______		
12	Did you ever have abortion?	1. Yes 2. No		
13	Para[Number of births]	1. Number of children alive______ 2. Number of children died_____ 3. Number of still birth______		
14	Did you ever have Problems in last delivery?	1. Yes 2. No		
15	Have you history of previous caesarean delivery?	1. Yes 2. No		

Section III knowledge of ANC

16.	How do you rate the importance of ANC for your health?	1. Highly important 2. medium 3. Less 4. Do not know		
17.	How do you rate the importance of ANC for your fetus?	1. Highly important 2. medium 3. Less 4. Do not know		
18.	When do you think it is appropriate time to begin the ANC after last menstrual period?	at_______months		
19.	How many times do you think a woman needs to go for ANC during pregnancy?	1. One Visit 2. Two times 3. Three times 4. More than four times		

Section IV past history of service utilization

20.	Have you ever attended ANC?	1. Yes 2. No ⟶	26	
21.	If yes to the above question for which Pregnancy you have attended?	1. 1st pregnancy 2. 2nd pregnancy 3. 3rd pregnancy 4. 4th pregnancy 5. 5th pregnancy		
22.	For your last pregnancy, when did you first go to the health facilities for antenatal care?	1 At_______months 2 I don't known		
23	Is there any payment you were asked for checkup?	1. Yes 2. No		

24	If yes for Q 23, for what services you paid?	1.For consultation [card and Examination] 2. For laboratory 3. For ultrasound 4. For drugs 5.Other[specify]____________		
25	If you paid for any service charge, what is the maximum money you paid for a visit?	1. less than or equal 10.00 ETB 2. 11.00 - 20.00 ETB 3. 21.00 – 50.00 ETB 4. Greater than 50.00 ETB		
26.	Rate the following items of service in terms of your satisfaction	1. Staff approach	1. Highly satisfied 2. Satisfied 3. Medium 4. Not satisfied 5. Highly not satisfied	
		2 laboratory	1. Highly satisfied 2. Satisfied 3. Medium 4. Not satisfied 5. Highly not satisfied	
		3.Waiting time	1. Highly satisfied 2. Satisfied 3. Medium 4. Not satisfied 5. Highly not satisfied	
		4. Privacy	1. Highly satisfied 2. Satisfied 3. Medium 4. Not satisfied 5. Highly not satisfied	

Section V History of current pregnancy

27	How do you know your pregnancy?	Missed period once Missed period twice Missed period three and more Physiological changes Other signs like nausea By examination [urine test] Other [specify]____________		
28.	How many times did you receive antenatal care during this pregnancy?	1. It is my first time 2. Two times 3. Three times 4. Four times 5. Greater than four		
29.	Is this pregnancy planned?	1.yes 2. No →	30	
30.	If this pregnancy is planned, did the plan include your husband?	1.yes 2. No		
31.	If this pregnancy is not planned, was it wanted by you after conception?	1.yes 2. No		
32.	If this pregnancy is not planned was it wanted by your husband after conception?	1.yes 2. No		

Section VI History of current ANC

33.	Do you have problem in the current pregnancy?	1. Yes 2. No		
34.	Before your first attendance of the ANC, was there any one who advised you to come?	1. Yes 2. No		
35.	If yes for Q 33, to above question, from whom you get advice?	1. Community health workers 2. Husband 3. Mother 4. Sister 5. Friend 6.Other[specify]____________		
36.	In the present pregnancy, when did you start the follow up?	1. After ______months of amenorrhea 2. I don't know the exact months		
37.	Why you decide to start [begin] the follow up at this time?	1. Thought it was appropriate time 2. Delay due to finance 3. Booking at convenience 4. Given appointment for today 5. Delay due to time 6. Others[specify]______________		

This is all what I want to ask you. Thank you for spending your time and valuable information you gave us. Do you have any question that I can address for you?

____

____

____

Qualitative research tool

Focus group discussion and probes

1. How do you feel when you first knew that you were a pregnant?

   Probe: What kind of emotion did you have?

   What kind of symptoms did you have that made you realize you were pregnant?

   Did you discuss it with your family?

   What decision did you take about seeing a doctor?

2. What stopped you from starting after you found out you were pregnant?
3. When you knew you were pregnant how long did it take to be seen by health provider?

   Probe: Have you had any trouble being seen at the hospital/ health center?

   How do you feel about being pregnant?

   What are your thoughts on pregnancy?

4. Should a pregnant woman go and see health provider if she's not having any problems? Why? Why not?
5. Who do you have for social support?

   Probes: Family members, spouse, neighbors, friends, church members?

   Can you get any of them to help you go to your prenatal care appointment?

6. What do you think is the reasons that some women fail to book early in pregnancy?

Annex III Amharic Informed Consent Sheet

ጤና ይስጥልኝ፡፡ ስሜ-------------------------------ይባላል፡፡ በዚህ ሆስፒታል/ጤና ጣቢያ ውስጥ ነርስ/አዋላጅ ነርስ/ በመሆን እያገለገልኩ ነው፡፡ እንዲሁም ነፍሰጡር እናቶች ለምን ዘግይተው ቅድመ ወሊድ ክትትል ይጀምራሉ በሚል ላይ ጥናት ከሚያደርጉ ቡድን ጋ በመስራት ላይ እገኛለሁ፡፡

በአሁን ጊዜ እናቶች/ነፍሰጡር ለምን የቅድመ ወሊድ አገልግሎትን ዘግይተው ይጀምራሉ የሚል ምንያት ለመለየት ጥናት እያደረግን ነው፡፡ ለዚህም መረጃ በማሰባሰብ ላይ እንገኛለን፡፡ የዚህም ጥናት ዋናው ዓላማ ነፍሰጡር እናቶች ለምን የቅድመ ወሊድ አገልግሎትን ዘግይተው ይጀምሉ የሚለውን ምክንያቱን መለየት ሲሆን፣ ለእናቶችና ለሕፃናቶች የሚደረገውን እንክብካቤ ለማሻሻል ይረዳል ተብሎ ይታመናል፡፡ ስለዚህ በዚህ ጥናት እንዲሳተፉ እንጋብዞታለን፡፡

በጥና ላይ ተሳታፊ ከሆኑ ከ10-15 ደቂቃ ይወስድቦታል፡፡ የእርስዎ ስም በዚህ መጠይቅ ላይ አይሞላም፡፡ ስለዚህ የሚሰጡት መረጃ ሁሉ ሚስጢራዊነቱ እጅግ የተጠበቀ ይሆናል፡፡ ተሳትፎዎ ሙሉ በሙሉ በእርሶዎ ፈቃደኝነት ላይ ብቻ የተመሰረተ ይሆናል፡፡ እንዲሁም በፈለጉት ጊዜ ውይይቱን ማቋረጥ ይችላሉ፡፡ ባለመሳተፍዎ ወይም ውይይቱን በማቋረጥዎ ከሆስፒታሉ/ጤናጣቢያ ውስጥ የሚያገኙት አይጓደልቦትም፡፡ ይሁን እንጂ የእርስዎ ተሳትፎ በጣም አስፈላጊ በመሆኑ በጥናቱ እንዲሳተፉ ተስፋ እናደርጋለን፡፡

በቃለ መጠይቁ ለመሳተፍ ፈቃደኛ ነዎት?

ስለጥናቱ ጥያቄ ካለዎት ከዚህ በታች በተጠቀሰዉ አድራሻ ዋና ተመራማሪዉን ማግኘት ይቻላል፡፡

ስም ታሪኩ እንዳሻዉ አለሙ

አድራሻ አዲስ አበባ ዩኒቨርሲቲ , ህብረተሰብ ጤና ት/ት ክፍል

አዲስ አበባ, እትዮጵያ

የስልክ ቁጥር 0912-08-21-34

E- Mail endashawtariku@yahoo.com

አዲስ አበባ ዩኒቨርሲቲ, ህክምና ፋኩልቲ IRB

የስልክ ቁጥር 0115538734

E-Mail aaumfirb@yahoo.com

ለ. <u>የፍቃደኝነት ማረጋገጫ ቅፅ</u>

እኔ በጥናቱ ላይ እንድሳተፍ የተጠየቅኩ ከዚህ በላይ በጥናቱ መረጃ ቅፅ ላይ የተቀመጠዉን ነገር በአግባቡ በመረዳት ከእኔ የሚጠበቀዉን ሁሉ አዉቄያለሁ:: ከዚህም ሌላ በጥናቱ ላይ ተሳታፊ ቢሆን እኔ የምሰጣቸዉ መረጃዎች ለሶስተኛ አካል ተላልፈዉ እንደማይታወቁና የግለሰብ ስም እንደማይካተት ተረድቻለሁ::በተጨማሪም ጥናቱን የማልፈልገዉ ከሆነ በማንኛዉም ሰዓት ያለምንም ምክንያት ማቆም ወይም ማቆም እንደምችልና በማቆሜም እኔ ወይም በተሰቦቼ ከድርጅቱ በሚያገኙት አገልግሎት ላይ ምንም ዓይነት ተፅዕኖ እንደማይኖረዉ አዉቄያለሁ::

በቃለ መጠየቁ ለመሳተፍ ፈቃደኛ ነዎት?

በጥናቱ ለመሳተፍ

1. ተስማምተዋል ☐
2. አልተስማሙም ☐ → አመስግነህ/ሽ ጨርስ/ሺ

<u>የቃለ መጠየቅ አድራጊዉ/ ዋ ስምምነት</u>

ተሳታፊዋ በጥናቱ ላይ ለመሳተፍ ፍቃደኝነታን የሚገልፅ ስምምነት በፅሑፍ መልክ መዉሰዴንና ስምምነቱም ትክክለኛ መሆኑን እገልፃለሁኝ::

የቃለ መጠየቅ አድራጊዉ/ዋ ስም________________________________ፊርማ__________________

/___________________/_____________________/ 2010 ዓ.ም

ቀን ወር

የተቆጣጣሪዉ/ዋ ስም________________________________ ፊርማ__________________

/___________________/_____________________/ 2010 ዓ.ም

ቀን ወር

ስለጥናቱ ጥያቄ ካለዎት ከዚህ በታች በተጠቀሰዉ አድራሻ ዋና ተመራማሪዉን ማግኘት ይቻላል::

ስም ታሪኩ እንዳሻዉ አለሙ

አድራሻ አዲስ አበባ ዩኒቨርሲቲ , ህብረተሰብ ጤና ት/ት ክፍል

አዲስ አበባ, ኢትዮጵያ

የስልክ ቁጥር 0912-08-21-34

E- Mail endashawtariku@yahoo.com

አዲስ አበባ ዩኒቨርሲቲ, ህክምና ፋኩልቲ IRB

የስልክ ቁጥር 0115538734

E- Mail aaumfir@yahoo.com

Amharic Questionnaire

የእናትየዋ ኮድ........./________/________/	ቀን/________/_________/ 2010 ዓ.ም
የቃለ መጠየቅ አድራጊው/ዋ ስም_______________________	የቃለ መጠይቅ አድራጊው ኮድ........

ቃለመጠይቁ የተጀመረበት ሰዓት ------:------ ***የተጠናቀቀበት ሰዓት----:-----***

ተ.ቁ	ጥያቄዎች	መልስ	እለፊ/ፍ	ኮድ

ክፍል አንድ: ማህበራዊና ዲሞግራፊያዊ ሁኔታዎች

1	እድሜዎ ስንት ነው?	__________ዓመት		
2	ብሔርዎ ምንድነው?	1. አኝዋክ 2. ኑዌር 3. መዠንገር 4. አማራ 5. ኦሮሞ 6. ሌላ/ይገለፅ/__________		
3	የመኖሪያ አካባቢ የት ነው?	1. ገጠር 2. ከተማ		
4	ሐይማኖትዎ ምንድነው?	1. ኦርቶዶክስ 2. ፕሮቴስታንት 3. ሙስሊም 4. ካቶሊክ 5. ሌላ/ይገለጽ__________		
5	የጋብቻ ሁኔታዎ እንዴት ነው?	1. ፈፅሞ ያላገባ 2. ያገባና አሁን አብሮ የሚኖር 3. የፈታ 4. በሞት የተለየ		
6	ትምህርት ቤት ገብተው ተምረዋል?	1. አዎ 2. የለም →	8	
7	ያጠናቀቁት የመጨረሻ የት/ት ደረጃ ስንት ነው?	1. ክፍል__________ 2. የቴክኒክ/ሙያ ሰርተፊኬት 3. የዩኒቨርስቲ/ኮሌጅ ዲፕሎማ 4. የዩኒቨርስቲ/ኮሌጅ ድግሪ ወይም ከዚያ በላይ		
8	አሁን ምን ዓይነት ስራ ነው የሚሰሩት?	1. የመንግስት ሰራተኛ 2. የግል ተቀጣሪ 3. የቤት እመቤት 4. የግል ስራ 5. ግብርና 6. ሌላ/ይገለጽ________		

9	የቤተሰብዎ ወርሃዊ ገቢ ምን ያህል ነው?	በወር__________የኢ.ት.ብር		
10	ወደዚህ ጤና ድርጅት ደርሰው ለመመለስ የከፈሉት ትራንስፖርት ምን ያህል ነው?	1. ምንም አልከፈልኩም 2. __________የኢ.ብር		

ክፍል ሁለት: የእናትየዋ የወሊድ ታሪክ

11	የአሁኑን ፅንስ በመጨመር እስከ አሁን ስንት ጊዜ አርግዘዋል?	1__________		
12	ከዚህ በፊት ውርጃ አጋጥሞዎት ያውቃል?	1. አዎ 2. የለም		
13	እስከአሁን ስንት ልጆች አልዎት?	1. በሕይወት ያሉ ብዛት__________ 2. ከተወለዱ በኋላ የሞቱ ብዛት__________ 3. ሞተው የተወለዱ ብዛት__________		
14	በወሊድ ላይ ችግር አጋጥሞዎታል (የሚቀርበው ወሊድ)?	1. አዎ 2. የለም		
15	ከዚህ በፊት በቀዶ ጥገና ሕክምና ወልደው ያውቃሉ?	1. አዎ 2. የለም		

ክፍል ሶስት: የቅድመ ወሊድ ክትትል እውቀት

16	የቅድመ ወሊድ ምርመራ ለጤንነትዎ አስፈላጊነቱን እንዴት ይገነዘቡታል?	1. በጣም አስፈላጊ ነው 2. በመጠኑ አስፈላጊ ነው 3. በጣም አነስተኛ ነው		
17	የቅድመ ወሊድ ምርመራው በማህፀን ላለው ልጅ አስፈላጊነቱን እንዴት ይገነዘቡታል?	1. በጣም አስፈላጊ ነው 2. በጣም አስፈላጊ ነው 3. በጣም አነስተኛ ነው		
18	የነፍሰ ጡር የቅድመ ወሊድ ክትትል የወር አበባ ከቆመ በኋላ መቼ ብጀመር ጥሩ ነው ብለው ይገምታሉ?	1. __________ወር		
19	አንድ ነፍሰጡር እናት ስንት ጊዜ የቅድመ ወሊድ አገልግሎት ብታገኝ ጥሩ ነው ብለው ይገምታሉ?	1. አንድ ጊዜ ብቻ 2. ሁለት ጊዜ 3. ሶስት ጊዜ 4. ከአራት ጊዜ በላይ		

20	የቅድመ ወሊድ/የነፍሰ ጡር ምርመራ ተከታትለው ያውቃሉ?	1. አዎ 2. አላውቅም →		26	
21	የነፍሰ ጡር ምርመራ ተከታትለው የሚያውቁ ከሆነ ለየትኛው እርግዝና ነው የተከታተሉት?	1. የመጀመሪያ እርግዝና 2. ሁለተኛ እርግዝና 3. ሶስተኛ እርግዝና 4. አራተኛ እርግዝና			
22	ከዚህ እርግዝና በፊት የነበረው እርግዝና የቅድመ ወሊድ ተከታትሎ ከሆነ የወር አበባዎ ቀርቶ በስንተኛ ወር ነው?	____________ወር			
23	ለነፍሰ ጡር ቅድመ ወሊድ ምርመራ የከፈሉት ገንዘብ ነበረ?	1. አዎ 2. የለም			
24	ለጥያቄ 23, መልሶ አዎ ከሆነ ለምን ጉዳይ ነበር የከፈሉት?	1. ለመታየትና ለካድ 2. ለላቦራቶሪ 3. ለአልትራሳውንድ 4. ለመድሃኒት መግዣ 5. ሌላ/ይገለጽ__________			
25	ለነፍሰጡር ቅድመ ወሊድ ምርመራ የከፈሉት ገንዘብ ካለ በአንድ ምርመራ ከፍተኛው የከፈሉት ገንዘብ ምን ያህል ነበር?	1. ከ10 ብር በታች 2. ከ11-20 ብ 3. ከ21-50 ብ 4. ከ50 ብር በላይ			
26.	የሚከተሉትን የአገልግሎት አሰጣጥ በእርስዎ የእርካታ መጠን ይግለፁት	1. የባለሙያዎች አቀራረብ	1. በጣም ረኪቻለሁ 2. ረኪቻለሁ 3. መካከለኛ ነኝ 4. አልረካሁም 5. በጣም አልረካሁም		
		2. የላብራቶሪ ምርመራ	1. በጣም ረኪቻለሁ 2. ረኪቻለሁ 3. መካከለኛ ነኝ 4. አልረካሁም 5. በጣም አልረካሁም		
		3. ምርመራው የሚፈጀው ግዜ	1. በጣም ረኪቻለሁ 2. ረኪቻለሁ 3. መካከለኛ ነኝ 4. አልረካሁም 5. በጣም አልረካሁም		
		4. ገበና አጠባበቅ	1. በጣም ረኪቻለሁ 2. ረኪቻለሁ 3. መካከለኛ ነኝ 4. አልረካሁም 5. በጣም አልረካሁም		

ክፍል አምስት: የአሁን እርግዝና መረጃዎች

27	ማርገዝዎን በምን ነበር ያወቁት?	1. የወር አበባዬ መምጣት ከነበረበት በአንድ ወር በመዘግየቱ 2. የወር አበባዬ መምጣት ከነበረበት በሁለት ወራት በመዘግየቱ 3. የወር አበባዬ መምጣት ከነበረበት በሶስት ወራት እናት ከዚያም በላይ በመዘግየቱ 4. የሰውነት ለውጥ በራሴ ላይ ስላየሁኝ 5. የሰውነት ለውጥ በራሴ ላይ ስላየሁኝ 6. ማቅለሽለሽ እና የመሳሰሉ ምልክቶች በማየት 7. የሽንት ምርመራ ለማድረግ 8. በሌላም መንገድ ካለ/ ይገለፅ________		
28	በዚህኛው እርግዝና የቅድመ ወሊድ አገልግሎት ለስንት ያህል ጊዜ አግኝተሻል?	1. ይህ የመጀመሪያዬ ነው 2. ለሁለት ጊዜ 3. ለሶስት ጊዚያት 4. ለአራት ጊዜያት 5. ከአራት ጊዜያት በላይ		
29	ይህ እርግዝናዎ የታቀደ እርግዝና ነበር?	1. አዎ 2. አይደለም →	30	
30	ይህ እርግዝና የታቀደ ከሆነ እቅዱ ባለቤትዎን አካቷል?	1. አዎ 2. አይደለም		
31	ይህ እርግዝናዎ ያለእቅድ ከሆነ ከተረገዘ በኋላ በእርሳዎ ይፈለግ ነበር?	1. አዎ 2. አይደለም		
32	ይህ እርግዝናዎ ያለዕቅድ ከሆነ ከተረገዘ በኋላ በባለቤትዎ ይፈለግ ነበር?	1. አዎ 2. አይደለም		
33	በዚኛው እርግዝና ላይ ችግር አጋጥሞታል?	1. አዎን 2. የለም		
34	የቅድመ ወሊድ አገልግሎት ሳይጀምሩ በፊት ወደዚህ እንዲመጡ የመከረዎት ሰው ነበር?	1. አዎን 2. የለም		
35	የቅድመ ወሊድ /ነፍሰ ጡር/ ምርመራ አገልግሎት አስፈላጊነት ተመክረው ከሆነ ምክሩን የሰጠዎት ማነው?	1. የህብረተሰብ ጤና ሰራተኛ 2. ባለቤትዎ 3. እናትዎ 4. እህትዎ 5. ጓደኛ 6. ሌላ/ይገለፅ________		
36	በዚህኛው እርግዝና የቅድመ ወሊድ አገልግሎት መች ነበር የጀመሩት?	1. የወር አበባዬ ከቀረ ከ________ወር በኋላ 2. ጊዜውን በእርግጠኝነት አላውቅም	አመስግነህ /ሺ. ጨርስ/ሺ.	
37	በዚህ ጊዜ ምርመራ አድርጎ ክትትሉን ለመጀመር ለምን ነበር የወሰኑት?	1. ጊዜው እንደሆነ ስለተነገረኝ 2. ገንዘብ ስለቸገረኝ 3. ምቹ ጊዜ ስለሆነልኝ 4. ጊዜ ስላጠረኝ 5. ሌላ/ይገለፅ________		

ጊዜሽን ሰጪተሽ ለሰጠሽኝ መረጃ ከልብ እያመሰገንኩኝ በጥናቱ ላይ ግልፅ ያልሆነልሽ ነገር ካለ ልትጠይቂኝ ትችያለሽ።

____

____

____

የቡድን ውይይት ጥያቄዎች

1. መፀነስሽን ስታዊቂ ለመጀመሪያ ጊዜ የተሰማሽ ስሜት ምን ዓይነት ነበር?

    አብራራ/ሪ - ምን አይነት ስሜት/ሁኔታ?

    - የበለጠ መፀነስሽን ያረጋገጥሽው ምን ዓይነት ምልክቶችን በራስሽ ላይ ስታይ ነው?
    - ስለ ፅንሱ ከቤተሰቦችሽ ጋር ተወያይተሽልን?
    - ወደ ጤና ባለሙያ/ሐኪም ሄደሽ ለማማከር ምን እርምጃ ነበር የወሰድሽው?
2. መፀነስሽን ካረጋገጥሽ በኋላ የነፍሰጡር የቅድመ ወሊድ አገልግሎት እንዳትጀምሪ ያደረገሽ ነገር ምንድነው?
3. መፀነስሽን ካረጋገጥሽ በኋላ ሐኪም/ጤና ባለሙያ ጋር እስክትሄጂ ድረሽ ምን ያህል ጊዜ ነው የቆሽው? (የቅድመ ወሊድ አገልግሎት ሳትጀምሪ)

    አብራራ/ራ- በሐኪም/ጤና ባለሙያ ለመታየት የቆየሽበት ነገር ምንድነው?

    -ለፅንሱ ያለሽ አመለካከት ምን ይመስላል?
4. አንድ ነፍሰጡር እናት ምንም ዓይነት ችግር ባይገጥማትም ሐኪም /የጤና ባለሙያን ማማከር ይጠበቅባታል ብለሽ ታስቢያለሽ?

    ለምን?

    እንዴት?
5. እርዳታ ያደርጉልሽ ዘንድ በእርግዝናሽ ጊዜ ሰው ከጎንሽ አለሽ ወይ?

    አብራራ/ሪ - የቤተሰብ አባላት፣ጓደኛ፣ጎረቤት፣ሌላ

    - ከእነዚህ ሰዎች መካከል በቀጠሮሽ ቀን የቅድመ ወሊድ አገልግሎትን እንድታገኚ የሚረዳሽ ይኖራሉን?
6. አንዳንድ እናቶች የቅድመ ወሊድ ክትትልን በጊዜ አይጀምሩም ይህ ከምን የመነጨ ነዉ ብለዉ ይገምታሉ?

I declare that

Assessment of late entry to antenatal care and its predictors among ANC in Gambella Region, is my own work and that all the sources I have used or quoted have been indicated and acknowledged by means of complete reference.

Name Tariku Endeshaw

Signature ________________

Place Addis Ababa, Ethiopia

Date of Submission June, 2010.

This thesis work has been submitted for examination with my approval as university advisor.

Misganaw Fantahun ________________

Advisor's Name Signature

MIX
Papier aus verantwortungsvollen Quellen
Paper from responsible sources
FSC® C105338

Printed by Books on Demand GmbH, Norderstedt / Germany